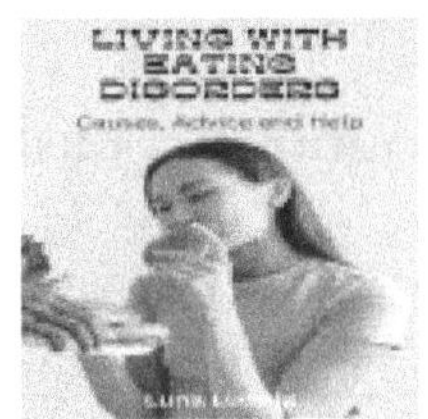
LIVING WITH
EATING
DISORDERS
Causes, Advice and Help

Introduction: What are eating disorders?

Eating disorders are mental illnesses characterized by abnormal eating behaviors and/or negative thoughts about food intake and body image. These disorders can take various forms, including anorexia (anorexia nervosa), bulimia (binge eating disorder) and binge eating disorder (binge eating). Anorexia is an eating disorder characterized by an unhealthy fear of gaining weight and inadequate food intake. People with anorexia often avoid foods they consider "fattening" and often eat extremely little food in order to lose weight or maintain their current weight. In severe cases, anorexia can lead to life-threatening complications such as dehydration, electrolyte imbalances and organ failure. Bulimia is an eating disorder characterized by recurrent episodes of uncontrollable eating followed by compensatory behaviors such as vomiting, abuse of laxatives or excessive exercise. People with bulimia often feel that they have no control over their eating behavior and may experience strong feelings of guilt and shame after a binge. Binge eating disorder is an eating disorder characterized by recurrent episodes of uncontrollable eating associated with feelings of guilt, shame and disgust. People with binge eating disorder often feel that they have no control over their eating habits and can feel isolated and alone because of their eating behavior. Binge eating disorders can occur at any age and in both genders, but are more common in women. They can be caused by a combination of factors, including genetic, biological, psychological and social factors. People with eating disorders may also struggle with other mental health conditions such as depression, anxiety and substance abuse. It is important to note that eating disorders are not a "choice" and are not caused by a lack of willpower or self-control. They are serious mental illnesses that require professional help. Without treatment, eating disorders can cause serious and life-threatening complications. In recent years, public awareness of eating disorders has increased and progress has been made in the research, treatment and prevention of these disorders. However, eating disorders remain a serious and often difficult-to-manage condition that affects many people. It is important that sufferers seek help early and contact a qualified professional to receive appropriate diagnosis and treatment.

History of eating disorders

How were they discovered and investigated? Eating disorders are mental disorders characterized by disordered eating behavior and/or body image. The most well-known eating disorders are anorexia nervosa, bulimia nervosa and binge eating disorder (BED). The history of eating disorders dates back to ancient times, but it took until the 20th century for them to be recognized as mental disorders in their own right. The first documented cases of eating disorders date back to antiquity. The Greek philosopher Plato described an eating disorder called "onania" (masturbation), in which people had to satisfy themselves before eating in order to suppress their appetite. Eating disorders such as anorexia nervosa were also documented in ancient Egypt and Rome. In the Middle Ages, eating disorders were regarded as religious asceticism and considered part of penance. In the 19th century, the French psychiatrist Ernest-Charles Lasègue described anorexia nervosa as a separate disorder for the first time and introduced the term "anorexia hystérique". In the 20th century, doctors and psychologists began to examine and define eating disorders in more detail. In 1927, the English doctor William Gull coined the term "anorexia nervosa" and described the symptoms and effects of the illness. In the 1930s, eating disorders were intensively studied by German doctors such as Franz Hildebrandt and Ludwig Knorr. They also coined the term "bulimia nervosa" and described the symptoms of this disorder for the first time. In the 1970s, anorexia nervosa was included as a separate diagnosis in the DSM (Diagnostic and Statistical Manual of Mental Disorders), which is published by the American Psychiatric Association (APA). In 1980, bulimia nervosa was included as a separate diagnosis in the DSM. Binge eating disorder (BED) was only later recognized as a separate diagnosis and added to the DSM in 2013. In recent decades, the understanding of eating disorders has evolved and various theories about their causes and treatment options have been proposed. One theory states that eating disorders are due to a combination of genetic, biological, psychological and social factors. Another theory is that eating disorders are influenced by cultural ideals and norms of body image, which can increase thinness and lead to a disturbed self-image. Today, there are various treatment options for eating disorders, including psychotherapy, medical treatment and support from self-help groups. However, treatment is often lengthy and requires a careful and holistic approach.

Types of eating disorders

Anorexia, bulimia, binge eating disorder and other eating disorders are serious mental illnesses associated with a disturbed relationship with food and one's own body. These disorders not only affect a person's physical health, but also their social and emotional well-being. The three main types of eating disorders, namely anorexia, bulimia and binge eating disorder, as well as some other eating disorders, are described below. Anorexia Anorexia is an eating disorder characterized by extreme weight loss and a severe fear of gaining weight. People with anorexia often have a distorted body image and see themselves as overweight when in fact they are underweight. They may drastically reduce their food intake, completely eliminate certain food groups or exercise excessively to burn calories. Anorexia can cause serious health problems, including heart problems, kidney failure, bone loss, infertility and even death. Treatment often involves a combination of psychotherapy, nutritional counseling and medication. Bulimia Bulimia is an eating disorder characterized by repeated episodes of binge eating followed by vomiting or the use of laxatives or diuretics to lose weight. People with bulimia often have a normal weight or are slightly overweight. They may also use other methods to burn calories, such as excessive exercise or fasting. Bulimia can lead to serious health problems, such as electrolyte imbalances, dehydration, damage to the esophagus and teeth, and stomach problems. Treatment often includes psychotherapy, nutritional counseling and medication. Binge eating disorder Binge eating disorder is an eating disorder characterized by repeated episodes of binge eating in which people consume large amounts of food in a short period of time even though they are not hungry. In contrast to bulimia, people with binge eating disorder do not usually take measures to lose weight, such as vomiting or using laxatives. This can lead to overweight or obesity. People with binge eating disorder may also suffer from depression, anxiety and low self-esteem. Treatment often includes psychotherapy, nutritional counseling and possibly medication. Orthorexia Orthorexia is an eating disorder in which people are overly concerned about what they eat and try to strictly adhere to a "healthy" diet.

Risk factors for eating disorders

What can contribute to developing an eating disorder? Eating disorders are complex mental illnesses that can take various forms, including anorexia, bulimia and binge eating disorder. The causes of eating disorders are multifactorial and can include biological, psychological and sociocultural factors. Some of the risk factors for eating disorders are explained below: Biological factors: There is evidence that biological factors may play a role in the development of eating disorders. Studies have shown that changes in brain chemistry, particularly in relation to the neurotransmitter serotonin, can play a role in the development of eating disorders. There may also be a genetic predisposition to eating disorders, so a family history of eating disorders can increase the risk of developing an eating disorder yourself. Psychological factors: There are several psychological factors that can increase the risk of developing eating disorders. A negative body image and low self-esteem are common characteristics of people with eating disorders. Those affected may feel that they are only accepted and loved if they achieve certain body measurements or shapes. A tendency towards perfectionism and high performance standards can also increase the risk of eating disorders. Socio-cultural factors: The ideals of Western beauty standards, which are characterized by slim bodies, can increase the risk of eating disorders. Women in particular are often affected by these ideals and put themselves and others under a great deal of pressure to achieve certain body measurements or shapes. Social factors, such as the availability of food and diet products, can also increase the risk of eating disorders. Traumatic experiences: Traumatic experiences, especially in childhood, can increase the risk of eating disorders. For example, one study found that people who had experienced childhood sexual abuse had a higher risk of eating disorders. Emotional neglect or maltreatment can also increase the risk of eating disorders. Dieting and excessive exercise: Dieting and excessive exercise can increase the risk for eating disorders. Many people start dieting or exercise excessively to lose weight or improve their body image. However, when these measures get out of control and end in an obsession with food and body image, this can manifest in an eating disorder. Stress: Stress can also increase the risk of eating disorders.

Prevention of eating disorders

How can you prevent it? Eating disorders are mental illnesses that are characterized by disturbed eating behavior. Those affected have a distorted perception of their body and their eating behavior and often develop an unhealthy relationship with food. Eating disorders such as anorexia, bulimia and binge eating can have serious physical and psychological consequences, including malnutrition, lack of essential nutrients, physical weakness, depression and anxiety. Fortunately, there are many ways to prevent binge eating. Here are some tips that can help promote healthy eating behaviors and a positive body image: Promote a positive body image: a healthy self-image and positive body image are critical to preventing eating disorders. Parents and guardians can help their children develop a positive body image by teaching them that every body is unique and that it is important to accept and appreciate their own body. Encourage healthy eating habits: Parents and guardians can teach children that it is important to have a balanced diet and eat regularly to provide the body with adequate nutrients. Children should also learn to listen to their bodies and only eat when they are hungry. Avoid body comparisons: Body comparisons with other people can lead to a negative self-image and increase the risk of eating disorders. It is important to teach children that every body is different and that it is not useful to compare themselves to others. Encourage exercise: Regular exercise is important for health and can help promote a positive body image. However, children should learn that exercise is not a means to lose weight and that it is more important to have fun and stay active. Avoid dieting: Dieting can lead to disordered eating behaviors and increase the risk of eating disorders. Parents and guardians should teach their children that it is important to have a balanced diet and not to focus on dieting. Be vigilant: Parents and guardians should look out for signs of eating disorders in their children, such as unusual eating habits, weight loss or gain, lack of energy and difficulty concentrating. If you have concerns, you should consult a doctor or therapist. Be a good role model: Parents and guardians should set a good example of healthy eating behavior.

Diagnosis of eating disorders

How are they diagnosed? Eating disorders are complex psychological disorders characterized by impaired eating behavior patterns and body image perceptions. The three most common eating disorders are anorexia nervosa (anorexia nervosa), bulimia nervosa (binge eating disorder) and binge eating disorder (binge eating). The diagnosis of eating disorders requires a comprehensive assessment of the patient's eating habits, physical symptoms and psychological states. Below you will find a summary of the diagnostic procedures for the various eating disorders: Anorexia nervosa Anorexia nervosa is diagnosed using criteria listed in the Diagnostic and Statistical Manual of Mental Disorders (DSM-5). Some of the most important criteria are: Significant weight loss resulting in a body weight at least 15% below expected or a body mass index (BMI) of 17.5 or below. A disturbed self-perception of one's own body image or a constant urge to reduce body weight or body measurements. A pronounced fear of gaining weight, which often leads to restrictive eating habits. Disorders in the hormonal system, such as amenorrhea (absence of menstruation) in women. To make a diagnosis of anorexia nervosa, at least three of the above criteria must be met. A doctor or therapist will also perform a physical examination to check for physical symptoms such as a drop in blood pressure, bradycardia (low pulse) and dehydration. Bulimia nervosa The diagnosis of bulimia nervosa is also based on the criteria listed in the DSM-5. Some of the most important criteria are Repeated episodes of binge eating, where a large amount of food is consumed in a short period of time, along with a sense of loss of control. Complex behavioral patterns to avoid weight gain, such as vomiting, excessive exercise, fasting or abuse of laxatives. Symptoms occur at least once a week for three months. A disturbed self-perception of one's own body image. To make a diagnosis of bulimia nervosa, at least three of the above criteria must be met. A doctor or therapist will also perform a physical examination to check for physical symptoms such as dental damage, dehydration and electrolyte imbalances. Binge Eating Disorder Binge eating disorder is also diagnosed based on criteria listed in the DSM-5.

Symptoms of anorexia

What are the signs of anorexia? Anorexia, also known as anorexia nervosa, is an eating disorder characterized by excessive weight loss, disturbed body image, and obsessive control of eating behavior. The symptoms of anorexia can have both physical and psychological effects and can occur in people of any age, gender or background. The following are some of the most common signs and symptoms of anorexia: Weight loss: a person with anorexia will often experience significant weight loss caused by a low calorie diet and excessive physical activity. Physical changes: Anorexia can lead to physical changes such as dry skin, brittle nails and hair, sensitivity to cold, muscle weakness and bone loss. Eating behavior: Individuals with anorexia may avoid certain food groups, consume excessive amounts of water or caffeinated beverages, or skip meals. Controlling behavior: People with anorexia often have a strong desire to control their food intake by measuring portion sizes or counting calories. Body image: People with anorexia may have impaired body image and misjudge their own body size and weight. Social isolation: People with anorexia may withdraw from friends and family and avoid social activities. Mood changes: Anorexia can lead to mood changes such as depression, anxiety and irritability. Physical illnesses: Anorexia can lead to a number of physical illnesses, including heart problems, kidney failure and hormonal imbalances. Eating disorder symptoms: People with anorexia may also have other eating disorder symptoms, such as bulimia or binge eating disorder. Addictive behaviors: People with anorexia may develop addictive behaviors toward controlling food and weight and may have difficulty stopping. It is important to note that not all people with anorexia have all of these symptoms. Some people may only have a few symptoms, while others may have several symptoms at the same time.

Causes of anorexia

Why do some people develop anorexia? Anorexia, also known as anorexia nervosa, is an eating disorder characterized by an obsessive desire to lose weight and a disturbed body image. It is a complex disorder caused by a combination of genetic, psychological, social and environmental factors. This text examines the most common causes of anorexia. Genetic factors Studies have shown that anorexia runs in families and that a person has a higher risk of developing the disorder if a family member is also affected. There is also evidence that certain genes associated with the regulation of mood, anxiety and appetite may increase the risk of developing anorexia. Psychological factors People who suffer from anorexia often have a disturbed body image and tend to monitor and evaluate their weight and figure excessively. They often set unrealistic weight loss goals and put themselves under pressure to achieve these goals. In addition, people with anorexia often have low self-esteem, perfectionism and a tendency towards compulsive behavior. Social factors Social factors, such as cultural pressure to be thin, can also play a role in the development of anorexia. In Western societies in particular, thinness is often associated with beauty, health and success. People who develop anorexia may try to live up to these social expectations by reducing their weight. Environmental factors Environmental factors, such as traumatic experiences, stress and life changes, can also contribute to the development of anorexia. People who have had a difficult childhood or experienced traumatic events may be more susceptible to developing anorexia. Stress and life changes can also increase the risk, as they can exacerbate the sense of loss of control that is often present in people with anorexia. Biological factors There is also evidence that biological factors, such as hormone imbalances, may play a role in the development of anorexia. In particular, the hormone leptin, which regulates appetite, has been linked to anorexia. People with anorexia have often been found to have low leptin levels. Summary Anorexia is a complex disorder caused by a combination of genetic, psychological, social and environmental factors. People who suffer from anorexia often have a disturbed body image.

Treatment of anorexia: How is anorexia treated?

Anorexia, also known as anorexia nervosa, is an eating disorder characterized by an excessive obsession with avoiding food and losing weight. Treatment for anorexia can be complex and lengthy, and usually requires a combination of medical treatment, psychotherapeutic interventions and support from family and friends. An important component of anorexia treatment is medical stabilization. Individuals with anorexia can have serious health problems due to food refusal and weight loss, such as electrolyte imbalances, heart problems, bone loss and organ failure. In the initial stages of treatment, medical monitoring may be necessary to ensure that the individual is stabilized and does not require acute emergency medical care. In addition to medical treatment, psychotherapy is an essential part of the treatment of anorexia. Psychotherapy aims to identify and treat the psychological problems and thought patterns that contribute to the development and maintenance of anorexia. One form of psychotherapy that is widely used for the treatment of anorexia is cognitive behavioral therapy (CBT). In CBT, individuals learn to identify their thought patterns and behaviors that contribute to anorexia and learn to develop new skills and strategies to make healthier choices about food and body weight. Another important component of anorexia treatment is nutritional counseling. Because anorexia is often associated with an excessive obsession with food and weight loss, people with anorexia may have difficulty regaining normal and healthy eating habits. A dietitian can help plan a balanced and healthy diet that is tailored to the specific needs of the individual while helping to build a healthy relationship with food and body weight. In addition to medical treatment, psychotherapy and nutritional counseling, support from family and friends is important. People with anorexia can feel isolated and have difficulty finding support and understanding from others. Relatives and friends can play an important role by providing emotional support, helping the individual to access medical and therapeutic care, and supporting them to regain healthy eating habits and behaviors. In some cases, inpatient treatment in a clinic or hospital may be necessary.

Symptoms of bulimia nervosa

What are the signs of bulimia? Bulimia is an eating disorder in which people regularly consume large amounts of food and then try to compensate for the calories by vomiting, excessive exercise or other methods of weight loss. Here are some common symptoms of bulimia: Binge eating: People with bulimia often have binge eating episodes where they consume large amounts of food in a short period of time, often without having control over what or how much they eat. Loss of control: During a binge eating episode, people with bulimia often feel helpless and out of control, which can lead to feelings of shame and guilt. Vomiting: A common method of compensating for binge eating in bulimia is vomiting, often by triggering the gag reflex. Laxative abuse: Another way to compensate for binge eating in bulimia is to abuse laxatives or other weight loss medications. Excessive exercise: People with bulimia tend to use excessive physical activity as a method of compensating for binge eating. Hidden binge eating: People with bulimia may hide binge eating by eating alone or in the absence of others. Weight problems: Bulimia can cause people with the disorder to have a normal body weight or even be overweight, although they may perceive themselves as obese. Body image issues: People with bulimia often have negative thoughts and feelings about their appearance and body shape, and their perception of their body is often distorted. Behavioral changes:

People with bulimia can often become withdrawn and socially isolated, and their moods can fluctuate wildly. Health problems: Bulimia can lead to a variety of physical and mental health problems, including dehydration, electrolyte imbalances, dental problems, digestive disorders and depression. It is important to note that not all people with bulimia have all of these symptoms, and the presence of only one or two symptoms does not necessarily mean that someone has bulimia. A diagnosis of bulimia requires a thorough assessment by an experienced professional in the field of eating disorders. If you or someone you know is showing symptoms of bulimia, it is important to seek help immediately. Treatment for bulimia may include a combination of psychotherapy, medical monitoring and nutritional counseling. With early detection and appropriate treatment, bulimia can be treated and a healthy life can be restored.

Causes of bulimia

Why do some people develop bulimia? Bulimia is an eating disorder in which people have repeated binge eating episodes and then try to compensate for the food they have eaten through various methods such as vomiting, abusing laxatives or exercising excessively. This disorder can have serious physical and psychological effects and is often a challenge for sufferers and their loved ones. The causes of bulimia are complex and can vary from person to person. However, there are some factors that can increase the risk of developing bulimia. Some possible causes of bulimia are explained below: Genetics: There is evidence that the predisposition to eating disorders such as bulimia may be due to genetic factors. Studies have shown that people whose parents or siblings suffer from bulimia or other eating disorders have a higher risk of developing bulimia themselves. Psychological factors: People with bulimia often have a history of mental health problems such as depression, anxiety or low self-esteem. These factors can contribute to those affected feeling dissatisfied with their body and weight, which in turn can lead to binge eating and other unhealthy behaviors. Societal factors: The pressure to be thin and conform to a certain ideal of beauty can make people more susceptible to eating disorders such as bulimia. Media and social networks can often show images of thin people, increasing the pressure to conform to a certain body image. Traumatic experiences: Some studies have shown that people who have experienced traumatic events such as abuse or neglect have a higher risk of developing eating disorders such as bulimia. Traumatic events can cause sufferers to develop unhealthy coping mechanisms such as binge eating and vomiting. Biological factors: Hormonal changes during puberty or related to the menstrual cycle can lead to binge eating in some women. Metabolic disorders or other physical illnesses can also promote the development of bulimia. It is important to note that there is not always a clear cause of bulimia and that many factors can combine to contribute to the development of the disorder. People with bulimia often require professional treatment to alleviate their symptoms and treat the underlying causes. Treatment for bulimia usually involves a combination of psychotherapy and medical care. Therapy can help treat the underlying psychological issues.

Treatment of bulimia How is bulimia treated?

Bulimia is a psychological disorder characterized by repeated binge eating followed by vomiting or the use of laxatives or diuretics. Treatment for bulimia usually involves a combination of psychotherapy and medication. Psychotherapy is an important component of bulimia treatment. One type of psychotherapy that is often used is cognitive behavioral therapy (CBT). CBT involves identifying and changing the thoughts and behaviors that lead to binge eating. It is also aimed at improving self-esteem and body image. Another form of psychotherapy that can be helpful is Interpersonal Psychotherapy (IPT). IPT aims to resolve relationship problems and reduce stress related to interpersonal relationships. Medication can also be part of the treatment for bulimia. Antidepressants such as SSRIs (selective serotonin reuptake inhibitors) can help to stabilize mood and reduce the frequency of binge eating. Some other medications such as antipsychotics can be used for more severe cases of bulimia. Another important component of bulimia treatment is nutritional counseling. A balanced diet can help minimize the physical effects of eating disorders while improving mood and overall well-being. A dietitian can also help establish healthy eating habits and show sufferers how to adjust their diet to compensate for nutritional deficiencies. Another important support for people with bulimia is a supportive community. Support groups such as Overeaters Anonymous can help build a supportive social network and connect with other people going through similar experiences. Family members and friends can also play an important role in supporting people with bulimia by providing emotional support and helping them to sustain their treatment. It is also important to emphasize that bulimia treatment can be a long-term process and that relapses can occur during the treatment process. Therefore, it is important that people with bulimia engage in a long-term treatment plan that addresses their needs and provides them with the support they require. Overall, treatment for bulimia requires a comprehensive approach that includes a combination of psychotherapy, medication, nutritional counseling and community support.

Symptoms of binge eating disorder

What are the signs of binge eating disorder? Binge eating disorder (BES) is an eating disorder characterized by recurring episodes of overeating accompanied by a sense of loss of control and feelings of shame. People with BES often have difficulty controlling their eating behavior and often eat large amounts of food even when they are not hungry. BES can lead to a range of physical, psychological and social problems. The following are some common signs of BES. Overeating: BES is characterized by overeating, in which the sufferer consumes large amounts of food in a short period of time. The sufferer often feels uncomfortably full and unwell after these episodes. Loss of control: People with BES often have the feeling of losing control over their eating behavior. They may feel that they cannot stop eating, even when they are full or feel uncomfortable. They may also feel that they cannot change their eating habits, even if they try. Secrecy: Those affected may hide their eating behavior and eat in secret to avoid others seeing how much they eat or to avoid feeling ashamed of their eating behavior. Guilt and shame: People with BES may feel guilty and ashamed of their eating behavior. They may judge themselves for their eating habits and feel ashamed of their body weight or appearance. Eating as a coping mechanism: Often people with BES use eating as a coping mechanism to deal with stressful or emotional situations. They may use eating as a way to protect themselves from problems or emotions. Thoughts about food: Sufferers may think about food frequently and spend excessive amounts of time thinking about food.

Causes of binge eating disorder

Why do some people develop binge eating disorder? Binge eating disorder (BED) is an eating disorder in which sufferers regularly consume large amounts of food in a short period of time, accompanied by the feeling of having lost control over their eating behavior. These binge eating episodes occur at least once a week for a period of three months and can lead to significant distress. Some of the causes of binge eating disorder are explained below: Psychological factors Psychological factors are often an important factor in the development of binge eating disorder. A variety of factors such as stress, anxiety, depression, low self-esteem, negative self-perception and emotional instability can cause people to develop unhealthy eating habits. Those affected often use eating as a coping mechanism to deal with stressful emotions. Binge eating can also be perceived as a form of "self-punishment" for perceived failure, guilt or shame. Biological factors There is evidence that biological factors play a role in the development of binge eating disorder. Research shows that people with BES have changes in their hormone balance that influence appetite and eating behavior. In particular, the hormone ghrelin, which indicates the feeling of hunger, appears to be higher in those affected, which can lead to an increased appetite and increased food intake. Social factors Social factors can also contribute to the development of binge eating disorders. Negative experiences such as bullying, exclusion or abuse can lead to people developing a disturbed relationship with their body and their eating behavior. Social pressure, particularly in relation to beauty ideals, can also lead to disordered eating behavior. Diets Diets that focus on strict calorie reduction or the avoidance of certain food groups can lead to people falling into a binge-eating spiral. Avoiding certain food groups can cause the body to crave them more and lead to cravings that can degenerate into binge eating. In addition, dieting can also lead to increased stress levels, which increases the risk of binge eating. Genetic factors There is also evidence that genetic factors can play a role in the development of binge eating disorders. Studies have shown that sufferers may have a higher genetic predisposition to eating disorders than those who are not affected.

Treatment of binge eating disorder

How is binge eating disorder treated? Binge eating disorder (BES) is an eating disorder in which people repeatedly consume large amounts of food in a short period of time and feel like they are losing control of their eating behavior. Binge eating disorder can lead to various health problems, including overweight, obesity, diabetes and high blood pressure. Treating binge eating disorder requires a comprehensive approach that addresses both physical and psychological aspects. This article discusses different approaches to treating binge eating disorder. Psychotherapy Psychotherapy is one of the most commonly recommended treatments for binge eating disorder. There are different types of psychotherapy that can be used, including cognitive behavioral therapy (CBT), interpersonal psychotherapy (IPT), psychodynamic psychotherapy, and group therapy. These therapies can help to identify and manage the underlying psychological issues and causes of binge eating disorder, such as anxiety, depression or stress. Cognitive behavioral therapy (CBT) is a widely used method for treating binge eating disorder. In CBT, patients work with a therapist to examine their thoughts, feelings and behaviors related to their eating behavior. The therapist helps the patient identify and change negative thoughts and behaviors. CBT can also help improve stress management skills and coping with negative emotions. Interpersonal psychotherapy (IPT) can also help in the treatment of binge eating disorder. This type of psychotherapy focuses on identifying and improving relationship problems and communication patterns that can contribute to maintaining binge-eating behaviors. IPT can also help improve self-esteem and problem-solving skills. Group therapy can also be helpful in treating binge eating disorder. Group therapy provides a supportive environment where patients can share their experiences and challenges with others who have had similar experiences. Group therapy can also provide an opportunity to learn from others and motivate each other. Medications Although there are no specific medications to treat binge eating disorder, some medications can be used to treat certain symptoms associated with the disorder. Antidepressants, particularly selective serotonin reuptake inhibitors (SSRIs), can help alleviate symptoms such as depression, anxiety and obsessive-compulsive disorder.

Eating disorders in children and adolescents

How do they differ from eating disorders in adults? Eating disorders are mental illnesses characterized by disordered eating behavior and an exaggerated preoccupation with one's own body weight and appearance. Eating disorders can affect people of all ages, but children and adolescents are particularly at risk. There are different types of eating disorders, such as anorexia, bulimia and binge eating disorder. Eating disorders can cause serious physical and psychological problems and therefore need to be recognized and treated early. Although eating disorders in children and adolescents can have similar characteristics to those in adults, there are also differences. Here are some of the most important differences: Causes: Eating disorders in children and adolescents can be triggered by a variety of factors, including genetic predisposition, personality traits, family problems, trauma and social influences. In contrast, eating disorders in adults are more often linked to cultural and social factors, such as the pressure to conform to a certain ideal of beauty or stress at work. Symptoms: Eating disorders in children and adolescents can manifest themselves differently than in adults. For example, children and adolescents with eating disorders may have difficulty accepting their weight and appearance and may feel anxious about their growth and physical development. They may also be anxious or depressed and have difficulty concentrating on their school or hobbies. In adults, symptoms are more often focused on food intake and body weight. Diagnosis: Diagnosing eating disorders in children and adolescents can be more difficult than in adults, as their body weight and physical development are still growing and therefore an individual assessment of weight is necessary. In addition, it can be difficult to distinguish between normal weight loss during growth and an eating disorder. A careful clinical assessment, including a detailed medical history and physical examination, is therefore of great importance. Treatment of eating disorders in children and adolescents may differ from treatment in adults. Children and adolescents may require multidisciplinary treatment, including medical monitoring, nutritional counseling and psychotherapy. Parents and family members may also be involved in treatment to provide support and information to promote the healing process. In contrast, adults may benefit from more focused psychotherapy and possibly medication.

Eating disorders and gender

How do they differ in women and men? Eating disorders are serious psychological disorders characterized by disordered eating habits and an unhealthy body image. Although eating disorders can occur in women and men, there are differences in the way they manifest themselves. In this article, I will provide an overview of how eating disorders differ in women and men and which gender-specific factors play a role. Anorexia nervosa (anorexia nervosa) is an eating disorder characterized by an intense desire to lose weight. People with anorexia nervosa often have a distorted perception of their body and believe that they are overweight when in fact they are underweight. Anorexia nervosa is more common in women than in men. Women are often more body conscious and are subject to greater social pressure to be slim. Women may also be biologically more susceptible to anorexia nervosa, as low estrogen levels have been linked to an increased risk of developing anorexia nervosa. Anorexia nervosa is less common in men, but when it does occur, it can be more severe. Men with anorexia nervosa often have a higher body mass index (BMI) than women with the disorder and may wait longer to seek help. Men with anorexia nervosa may also be more likely to be overlooked or stigmatized, as eating disorders are often seen as a "woman's disease." Bulimia nervosa (binge eating disorder) is an eating disorder characterized by repeated binge eating followed by vomiting or excessive exercise. Women have a higher risk of bulimia nervosa than men. The reasons for this may be similar to anorexia nervosa, including higher cultural expectations for women to be thin and biological factors such as hormonal changes. In men, the symptoms of bulimia nervosa may be more subtle and less obvious than in women. Men with bulimia nervosa often have a normal body weight or are overweight and may exercise more to control their weight. Men with bulimia nervosa may also be less likely to seek help or undergo treatment due to the belief that eating disorders are a "women's problem". Binge eating disorder is an eating disorder characterized by regular episodes of binge eating without subsequent vomiting or excessive exercise. Women have a higher risk of binge eating disorder than men. Binge eating disorders can be associated with depression, anxiety and other mental disorders, which are more common in women than in men.

Eating disorders and culture

How do they differ in different cultures? Eating disorders are mental disorders characterized by abnormal eating behavior and a disturbed perception of one's own body. These disorders can manifest and affect different cultures in different ways. In Western cultures, the ideology of beauty is often associated with a slim body, which can lead people, especially women, to develop an exaggerated concern about their weight. As a result, eating disorders such as anorexia and bulimia are more common in these cultures. Sufferers often try to control their weight by starving themselves, exercising excessively or overeating and then vomiting. However, it is important to note that eating disorders are not exclusive to Western cultures, but can also occur in other cultures. In some Asian countries, such as Japan and Korea, the ideal of beauty may be a slim body, but a pale complexion and small jawline are also considered aesthetically pleasing. These idealized beauty standards can cause people in these cultures to develop disordered eating behaviors. In Japan, for example, there is an eating disorder called "pica", where people eat inedible objects such as soil or sand in order to lose weight. Another example is the "slimming tea" culture in some Asian countries, where special types of tea are advertised to help people lose weight. In other cultures, eating disorders can also take different forms. In some African countries, for example, "fattening farms" can be a practice where young women are forced to eat unhealthy amounts of food in order to gain weight and be seen as more attractive. In some Latin American countries, there is also a tradition called "La Cuarentena", where women stay at home after the birth of their child and eat excessively and unhealthily during this time in order to regain their strength. It is important to emphasize that eating disorders in any culture can have a serious impact on those affected. However, it is also important to recognize that cultural influences can play a role in how eating disorders are perceived, practiced and treated. In some cultures, it may be more difficult to diagnose and treat eating disorders, as they may not be recognized as a mental illness or may be stigmatized. In many cultures, it can also be difficult to talk openly about mental health, which can lead to people with eating disorders hiding their problems or not asking for help. It is important to consider cultural differences when it comes to the diagnosis and treatment of eating disorders.

Eating disorders and self-image

How do eating disorders affect self-image? Eating disorders are mental illnesses that affect eating behavior and the perception of one's own body. They can have a major impact on a person's self-image and self-esteem. In this text, I will explain how eating disorders can affect self-image. First of all, it is important to understand that eating disorders are often associated with a distorted body image. People with eating disorders often see their body differently than it actually looks. For example, they may perceive themselves as too fat when in fact they are underweight. This distortion can lead to a negative perception of their own body and therefore their self-image. A common eating disorder in which body image is distorted is anorexia nervosa. People with anorexia nervosa often have a distorted body image and consider themselves too fat, even though they are actually underweight. This distortion can lead to a negative self-perception, as they think that they are not thin enough to be accepted. This can lead to a decrease in self-esteem and affect self-image. Another eating disorder that can affect self-image is bulimia nervosa. People with bulimia nervosa often have a normal weight, but they may still perceive themselves as too fat. After an episode of binge eating, they try to get rid of the food by vomiting or taking laxatives. The feeling of losing control over their eating behavior can lead to a negative self-image and low self-esteem. Binge eating disorder is another eating disorder that can affect self-image. People with binge eating disorder are often overweight and struggle with binge eating. They may feel weak or out of control, which can lead to a negative self-image. They may also feel that they are not accepted if they are not thin, which can lead to low self-esteem. People with eating disorders may also have difficulty regulating their thoughts and feelings. They may feel that they are unable to control their thoughts and emotions, which can lead to a negative self-perception. They may perceive themselves as weak or incapable, which can affect their self-image. It is important to note that eating disorders can not only affect self-image, but can also have serious physical and psychological effects. It is important to seek appropriate treatment for eating disorders to minimize both the physical and psychological effects. Treatment for eating disorders can also help to improve self-image.

Eating disorders and mental illness

How are eating disorders related to other mental illnesses? Eating disorders are mental disorders that manifest themselves through a disturbed attitude towards food and a change in eating behavior. They can manifest themselves in various forms such as anorexia nervosa, bulimia nervosa, binge eating disorder or eating disorder not otherwise specified (EDNOS). Although eating disorders are usually seen as separate illnesses, there is a close relationship between eating disorders and other mental illnesses. Depression and anxiety disorders Depression and anxiety disorders are often associated with eating disorders. People with depression and anxiety disorders often have disturbed eating behavior, which can lead to an eating disorder. At the same time, an eating disorder can increase the risk of developing a depression or anxiety disorder. It is a kind of vicious circle in which the two disorders reinforce and exacerbate each other. Personality disorders People with personality disorders have a high risk of developing an eating disorder. The risk is particularly high in people with borderline personality disorder. In people with personality disorders, eating disorders can serve as a coping mechanism to deal with emotions and inner conflicts. The eating disorder can also be a way to increase self-esteem or maintain control over life. Post-traumatic stress disorder (PTSD) People who have had a traumatic experience have an increased risk of developing an eating disorder. An eating disorder can be a coping mechanism to deal with the effects of the trauma. It can also be a way to control or avoid the trauma by focusing on eating behaviors. In some cases, the eating disorder can also be part of post-traumatic stress disorder (PTSD). Addiction Eating disorders share many similarities with addictive disorders. Both disorders can be characterized by a lack of control and impulsive behavior. People with addictions can also have disordered eating behavior and develop an eating disorder as a result. At the same time, people with eating disorders may also suffer from other addictions, such as alcoholism or drug abuse. Schizophrenia Schizophrenia and eating disorders can be linked. Some studies have shown that people with schizophrenia have an increased risk of developing an eating disorder. Disordered eating behavior can also be a symptom of schizophrenia. It can be influenced by hallucinations or delusions that affect the perception of the body and food.

Eating disorders and physical health

How do eating disorders affect physical health? Eating disorders are mental illnesses characterized by unhealthy eating behaviors and a disturbed body image. There are different types of eating disorders, including anorexia nervosa (anorexia nervosa), bulimia nervosa (binge eating disorder) and binge eating disorder. Eating disorders can have a significant impact on physical health and cause long-term complications. In this article, we will take a closer look at the effects of eating disorders on physical health. Anorexia Nervosa People with anorexia nervosa have a disturbed body image and see themselves as too heavy, even though they are underweight. They eat very little or nothing at all and often try to lose weight by exercising excessively or taking laxatives. This type of eating disorder can lead to a number of health complications, including Malnutrition: when the body doesn't get enough nutrients, it can lead to a variety of problems, including weakness, fatigue, anemia, osteoporosis and muscle wasting. Cardiovascular problems: People with anorexia nervosa often have an irregular heartbeat and low blood pressure, which can lead to fainting, dizziness and heart problems. Hormonal changes: Inadequate nutrition can lead to hormone imbalances, especially in women, which can lead to infertility and menstrual problems. Bone problems: Malnutrition and weight loss can lead to bones becoming weaker and a higher risk of osteoporosis. Bulimia Nervosa (binge eating disorder) People with bulimia nervosa have recurring episodes of binge eating, where they eat large amounts of food, followed by behaviors to remove the food from the body, such as vomiting or abusing laxatives. Bulimia nervosa can lead to a number of health complications, including: Electrolyte imbalance: the constant vomiting can lead to a lack of electrolytes such as potassium, which can lead to heart problems, muscle cramps and kidney problems. Digestive problems: Frequent vomiting can damage the stomach and esophagus, leading to heartburn, reflux and stomach pain. Dental damage: Vomiting can also lead to tooth decay and gum disease. Hormonal changes: Similar to anorexia nervosa, hormonal changes can occur, which can lead to infertility and menstrual problems.

Eating disorders and sexuality

How do eating disorders affect sexuality? Eating disorders and sexuality are two complex issues that are often linked. Eating disorders can affect sexuality in different ways, both psychologically and physically. In this text, I will describe some of the most common ways in which eating disorders can affect sexuality. An eating disorder is a mental illness characterized by a disturbed perception of one's own body and eating behavior. The three most common eating disorders are anorexia nervosa (anorexia nervosa), bulimia nervosa (binge eating disorder) and binge eating disorder. Eating disorders can also be associated with other mental illnesses such as depression, anxiety and self-harm behavior. Eating disorders can affect sexuality in many ways, including: Body image: Eating disorders can lead to a disturbed body image, which can affect both self-esteem and sexuality. People with eating disorders may perceive themselves as unattractive or inadequate, which can make them feel sexually uncomfortable or undesirable. Libido: Eating disorders can also affect libido, especially in women. Reduced food intake can cause the body to produce fewer hormones that are important for sexual arousal, which can lead to a reduced libido. Physical symptoms: Eating disorders can also cause physical symptoms that can affect sexuality. For example, anorexia nervosa can lead to a reduction in vaginal lubrication, which can cause pain during sexual intercourse. Eating disorders can also lead to a reduction in breast size and a reduction in testosterone levels in men. Avoidance of intimacy: People with eating disorders may withdraw from intimacy and sexuality due to body image issues and feelings of shame. They may also try to avoid sexual encounters to avoid being confronted with their disordered eating behavior. Conditioned shame: Eating disorders can also cause people to develop a conditioning of shame around sexual experiences. For example, people with anorexia nervosa may feel that their body is not good enough and feel ashamed when they get naked or become sexually active. Weight fluctuations: Eating disorders can also lead to weight fluctuations, which can make people feel uncomfortable in their bodies and anxious about sexuality. For example, people with bulimia nervosa may have a fear of overeating and then vomiting, causing them to avoid sexual experiences.

Eating disorders and relationships

How do eating disorders affect relationships? Eating disorders are complex illnesses that can have an impact not only on physical health, but also on mental health and interpersonal relationships. The impact of eating disorders on relationships can be diverse, ranging from difficulties in the relationship to problems in the social environment. This text explains some of the most common effects of eating disorders on relationships. Trust issues Eating disorders can make it difficult for those affected to trust other people. This can lead to major challenges, especially in relationships. For example, if a person with an eating disorder is constantly monitored or criticized by their partner, this can lead to a breach of trust and put a strain on the relationship. Isolation and social isolation People with eating disorders tend to withdraw and feel isolated. This can lead to them having difficulty maintaining friendships or forming new relationships. In romantic relationships in particular, this can lead to conflict if the partner feels neglected or unappreciated. Lack of emotional availability Eating disorders can cause those affected to be emotionally distant and have difficulty expressing their feelings. This can lead to them being perceived as inaccessible or unapproachable in relationships. If one partner feels that the other is emotionally unavailable, this can lead to frustration or even a relationship crisis. Conflicts and disputes Eating disorders can also lead to conflicts and disputes in relationships. This can be the case, for example, if the partner tries to help the person with the eating disorder but feels that this help is inappropriate or abusive. Or if the person with the eating disorder feels that their partner does not understand or support them. Codependency Sometimes the relationship itself can become part of the problem if the partner of the person with the eating disorder is trapped in a codependent relationship. This means that the partner tends to be overly concerned with the other person's needs and neglect themselves. This can lead to the partner feeling burnt out or overwhelmed and having difficulty maintaining the relationship. Stigma and shame Eating disorders are often accompanied by stigma and shame. People with eating disorders may feel embarrassed or guilty and try to hide or deny their disorder. This can make it difficult for them to build or maintain relationships.

Eating disorders and pregnancy

How do eating disorders affect pregnancy? Eating disorders are serious illnesses that can have an impact on various aspects of human life, including pregnancy. The type and severity of the eating disorder can affect pregnancy in different ways. Some of the most common eating disorders and their effects on pregnancy are described below. Anorexia nervosa Anorexia nervosa is an eating disorder characterized by a severe fear of gaining weight and a disturbed body image. Women with anorexia nervosa often have an inadequate body mass index (BMI), which means that they are underweight. This can lead to various problems during pregnancy, including an increased risk of miscarriage, premature birth and low birth weight. Women with anorexia nervosa may also have difficulty consuming adequate amounts of nutrients during pregnancy, which can lead to malnutrition and other health problems. Bulimia nervosa Bulimia nervosa is an eating disorder characterized by repeated episodes of binge eating followed by vomiting or other methods of weight loss. Women with bulimia nervosa may be of normal weight or overweight, but they often have a disturbed body image and a fear of gaining weight. During pregnancy, bulimia nervosa can lead to an increased risk of miscarriage, premature birth and low birth weight. Women with bulimia nervosa may also have difficulty consuming adequate amounts of nutrients during pregnancy. Binge eating disorder Binge eating disorder is an eating disorder in which repeated episodes of binge eating occur in which large amounts of food are consumed in a short period of time without any weight loss behavior to follow. Women with binge eating disorder may be overweight or obese and often have a disturbed body image. During pregnancy, binge eating disorder can lead to an increased risk of gestational diabetes, high blood pressure and caesarean section. Women with binge eating disorder may also have difficulty consuming adequate amounts of nutrients during pregnancy. Orthorexia nervosa Orthorexia nervosa is an eating disorder characterized by obsessive healthy eating and a disturbed body image. Women with orthorexia nervosa may have a normal weight, but they often have difficulty consuming adequate amounts of nutrients during pregnancy. This can lead to malnutrition and other health problems.

Eating disorders and nutrition

How do eating disorders affect nutrition? Eating disorders can have a significant impact on nutrition as they affect eating behavior and attitudes towards food. There are different types of eating disorders, all of which can have different effects on diet. Here are some common eating disorders and how they can affect diet: Anorexia nervosa: In anorexia, people have a distorted body image and an excessive desire to lose weight. They often eat very little or nothing at all and may tend to completely avoid certain food groups such as carbohydrates or fats. This can lead to malnutrition and a lack of important nutrients such as protein, vitamins and minerals. People with anorexia can also suffer from osteoporosis, as their bones are weakened due to a lack of calcium and other important nutrients. Bulimia nervosa: In bulimia, people often have binge eating episodes where they consume large amounts of food in a short period of time. They often follow these binges with self-induced vomiting or excessive physical activity to control weight. This can lead to an irregular diet that lacks certain nutrients. It can also lead to dehydration and electrolyte imbalances, which can lead to serious health problems. Binge eating disorder: In binge eating disorder, people have binge eating episodes where they consume large amounts of food in a short period of time, but unlike bulimia, they do not follow these episodes with self-induced vomiting or excessive physical activity. This can lead to an irregular diet that lacks certain nutrients. It can also lead to overweight and obesity, which increases the risk of cardiovascular disease, diabetes and other health problems. Orthorexia nervosa: In orthorexia, people have excessive cravings for "healthy" foods and often avoid certain food groups that they consider "unhealthy". This can lead to an unbalanced diet as certain nutrients may be lacking. It can also lead to social isolation and anxiety disorders, as people with orthorexia often have difficulty eating outside of their own kitchen. Pica: With pica, people have an unusual desire to eat things that are not normally considered food, such as soil, clay or hair. This can lead to an unbalanced diet, as important nutrients may be missing. It can also lead to serious health problems.

Eating disorders and exercise

How do eating disorders affect physical activity? Eating disorders and physical activity are closely linked. Eating disorders can affect both the amount and type of physical activity. In this text, I will discuss the different types of eating disorders and how they can affect physical activity. Eating disorders are a group of mental illnesses characterized by abnormal eating habits and a disturbed relationship with body weight and shape. There are different types of eating disorders, such as anorexia, bulimia and binge eating disorder. Each of these disorders has different effects on physical activity. Anorexia People with anorexia have a disturbed relationship with their body weight and shape. They often have the goal of greatly reducing their weight or keeping it below a certain level. To achieve this, they drastically reduce their calorie intake and may also exercise excessively. This excessive physical activity can lead to a variety of health problems, including muscle weakness, fatigue and injury. It is also possible that people with anorexia may decrease their physical activity due to physical limitations caused by the decreased caloric intake. This can lead to a further decrease in muscle mass and a deterioration in physical health. Bulimia People with bulimia have repeated episodes of binge eating followed by behaviors aimed at reducing caloric intake, such as vomiting, abusing laxatives, or excessive physical activity. Excessive physical activity can serve to reduce the guilt and shame caused by binge eating. However, this activity can also lead to a deterioration in physical health, as it can lead to exhaustion and muscle injuries. In addition, the excessive physical activity in people with bulimia can lead to an increased risk of injury, especially if they suffer from exhaustion or overexert the body. Binge eating disorder People with binge eating disorder have repeated episodes of binge eating where they consume large amounts of food in a short period of time with no attempt to reduce calorie intake. Unlike bulimia, people with binge eating disorder do not engage in behaviors to reduce caloric intake. Although these people may be less physically active than people with anorexia or bulimia.

Eating disorders and social media

How does social media influence eating disorders? Eating disorders such as anorexia, bulimia and binge eating disorder affect millions of people worldwide. In recent years, many experts have raised concerns that social media may be increasing the prevalence of these disorders. Here are some ways social media can influence eating disorders. Body image distortion Social media is full of photos of "perfect" bodies and beauty standards that are often unrealistic and unattainable. This can lead to a distorted body image, with people comparing their own bodies to these idealized images and feeling negative. For people with eating disorders, this can be particularly dangerous as they are already prone to negative self-perceptions and tend to fixate on their weight and shape. Reinforcement of diet culture Social media is often full of diet tips, "healthy" foods and weight loss transformations. While healthy eating and physical activity are important, this content can lead to people becoming obsessed with their diet and trying extreme diets to achieve the body they see on Instagram. For people with eating disorders, this can become a reinforcer for their behavior as they already tend to obsessively monitor their food and weight. Promoting unhealthy behaviors There are numerous accounts on social media that promote unhealthy eating habits such as fasting, overexercising and vomiting. People with eating disorders may see these accounts as validation of their own behavior and find themselves in a community of people doing similar things. This can lead them to view their behavior as "normal" or "right" and reinforce their eating disorder. Cyberbullying Cyberbullying can also play a role in eating disorders. People with eating disorders can be bullied or attacked because of their appearance or weight. Social media can reinforce this by making it easier to leave anonymous comments or share images that hurt others. For people with eating disorders, this can lead to increased pressure to further disguise their behavior and become even more intense. Confirmation of eating disorders In some cases, social media can contribute to the confirmation of eating disorders. People with eating disorders may find themselves in a community of people who support and normalize their behaviors. This community can lead them to view their behavior as "right" or "good" and be unwilling to seek treatment. Overall, social media has the potential to increase the prevalence of eating disorders.

Eating disorders and stigmatization

How are people with eating disorders stigmatized - Eating disorders are complex mental illnesses that can manifest in various forms, such as anorexia nervosa, bulimia nervosa and binge eating disorder. These disorders affect not only the physical well-being, but also the mental and emotional well-being of the person affected. Unfortunately, people with eating disorders are often stigmatized and misunderstood. In this text, I will take a closer look at how people with eating disorders are stigmatized. Prejudices and stereotypes People with eating disorders are often seen by society as weak and out of control. The prejudice that those affected could simply "stop" if they only wanted to is unfortunately widespread. This view does not take into account the fact that eating disorders are deeply rooted mental illnesses that cannot simply be cured with an act of will. Shame and guilt People with eating disorders often feel guilty and ashamed of their behavior. They often feel isolated and alone, which can cause them to withdraw even more. This shame and guilt are often also the result of the stigmatization and prejudice they face from society. Discrimination People with eating disorders can be discriminated against because of their illness. For example, they may have difficulties taking out health insurance or getting a job. People with eating disorders are often seen as unreliable and weak, which can lead to them being discriminated against because of their illness. Eating disorders are often trivialized or not taken seriously. This can lead to sufferers not receiving the support and treatment they need. It is important to understand that eating disorders are serious mental illnesses that need to be treated. Distorted portrayals in the media can also contribute to the stigmatization of eating disorders. Often, people with eating disorders are portrayed in the media as extremely thin and unhealthy, which can lead to the public having misconceptions about eating disorders.

Life after treatment

What happens after an eating disorder has been treated? Overcoming an eating disorder is a big step, but it's important to realize that recovery is a lifelong process. After treatment, there are many steps you can take to stay on the road to recovery. One option is to join a group of people who have also overcome or are working to overcome an eating disorder. These groups provide a way to connect with others who have had similar experiences and offer support and encouragement in times of relapse or challenge. An example of this is Overeaters Anonymous or Anorexics and Bulimics Anonymous meetings. It is also helpful to work with a therapist or counselor to respond to issues and receive support and guidance. A therapist can also help with learning and improving coping skills and tools to deal with stress, anxiety and other difficult emotions. Another important component of recovery is to maintain healthy eating habits. This means eating a regular, balanced diet to ensure adequate nutrient intake and maintain body weight. It can be helpful to work with a nutritionist to create an individualized meal plan and monitoring. Exercise is also an important part of life after eating disorder treatment, and it is important to find a healthy and sustainable form of exercise that does not trigger compulsivity. It is important to listen to your body and not overexert yourself. Self-care and stress management are also crucial to reduce the risk of relapse. Options include regular relaxation exercises such as yoga or meditation, participating in creative activities such as painting or writing, and setting up boundaries and priorities to minimize overwhelm and stress. The social environment is also an important factor in eating disorder recovery. Positive support and understanding from friends and family can be a great help, while negative or critical comments can increase the risk of relapse. It can be helpful to have a support group or partner to help you overcome challenges. It is important to note that recovery from eating disorders is an individual process, and everyone needs to find their own way. Relapses can happen, and it's important to accept them as part of the process and not get discouraged. Overall, eating disorder recovery can be a long and challenging process, but there are many resources and support options available to help with this.

Summary and outlook

Eating disorders are serious psychological disorders that affect a person's eating behavior and cause them to have a disturbed relationship with food and their own body. These include anorexia, bulimia and binge eating disorders. These eating disorders can have serious physical and psychological effects if left untreated. Summary: Anorexia, also known as anorexia nervosa, is an eating disorder characterized by a compulsive desire to lose weight. People with anorexia often have a distorted body image and see themselves as overweight when they are actually underweight. Treatment for anorexia involves a combination of psychotherapy, medical monitoring and nutritional therapy. Bulimia is an eating disorder characterized by repeated binge eating and a subsequent action to avoid gaining weight, such as vomiting or excessive physical activity. People with bulimia often have a normal body mass, but their eating behavior can still lead to serious physical and psychological problems. Treatment for bulimia involves a combination of psychotherapy and medical monitoring. Binge eating disorder (BED) is an eating disorder characterized by repeated binge eating episodes in which large amounts of food are consumed all at once. People with BED often have difficulty controlling their eating habits and feel guilty or ashamed afterwards. Treatment for BED involves a combination of psychotherapy and nutritional therapy. There are many risk factors that increase the risk of an eating disorder, such as genetic predisposition, mental illness and environmental factors such as social norms and beauty ideals. People with eating disorders need professional help to successfully treat their eating disorder. Outlook: Research into eating disorders has made progress in recent years and there are many new approaches to treating eating disorders. One promising method is cognitive behavioral therapy (CBT), which aims to change the behaviors and thought patterns that contribute to the eating disorder. There are also newer approaches such as Dialectical Behavior Therapy (DBT) and Acceptance and Commitment Therapy (ACT), which aim to help patients accept their thoughts and feelings and process them in a positive way. Another approach to treating eating disorders is the use of technology such as mobile apps and online programs to help people track their eating behaviors and moods and help them beat their disease.

Imprint

Luna Ludwig
Am Anger 3
06869 Coswig
Germany
Luna-Publishing.de